CONQUER YOUR DIET:

The Healthy Cookbook for a Family Eating Plan

Victor T. Rice

INTRODUCTION

Welcome to " Conquer Your Diet: The Healthy Cookbook for a Family Eating Plan"!

In today's fast-paced world, juggling the demands of work, family, and various commitments often leads to compromised meal choices and unhealthy eating habits. This book is a guide, a companion for families striving to prioritize health without sacrificing flavor or convenience in their meals.

Why Healthy Eating Matters for Families

We understand the challenges that come with ensuring our loved ones eat well. The importance of healthy eating extends beyond physical health; it influences our energy levels, mental well-being, and overall quality of life. In this book, we delve into the significance of balanced nutrition, offering insights into how it impacts each family member's growth, development, and daily performance.

How This Book Can Help You

Our aim is to simplify the process of preparing wholesome meals for your family. Throughout these pages, you'll discover practical tips, easy-to-follow recipes, and strategies for meal planning that align with busy lifestyles. We believe that with the right tools and knowledge, anyone can create delicious, nutritious meals that cater to diverse tastes and dietary preferences. From breakfast ideas that kick start your day to satisfying desserts that won't derail your health goals, each section of this book is curated to support your journey toward a healthier family eating plan. Our hope is that this book serves as a valuable resource, empowering you to make informed choices and transform the way your family views food.

Join us on this culinary adventure as we explore the world of nutritious, flavorful dishes and embark on a path toward wellness and vitality for you and your loved ones.

CHAPTER 1

FOUNDATIONS OF HEALTHY EATING

Healthy eating isn't just a trend; it's the cornerstone of a vibrant and balanced life for you and your family. In this chapter, we'll explore the fundamental principles that form the bedrock of a nutritious eating plan.

1. Understanding Macronutrients

a. Carbohydrates, Proteins, and Fats

We'll delve into the essential macronutrients, exploring their roles in the body, the right sources, and how to balance them in your meals for sustained energy and overall health.

b. Importance of Portion Control

Discover the significance of portion sizes and how they contribute to maintaining a healthy weight and supporting your family's nutritional needs.

2. Making Smart Food Choices

a. Whole Foods vs. Processed Foods

Learn how to differentiate between whole foods and processed options and why prioritizing whole, natural ingredients is beneficial for your family's well-being.

b. Reading Labels and Identifying Nutrient-Dense Foods

We'll discuss how to navigate food labels effectively, enabling you to select nutrient-dense foods and make informed choices while grocery shopping.

3. Balancing Variety and Moderation

a. Importance of a Varied Diet

Explore the benefits of incorporating a wide range of foods into your family's meals, ensuring they receive a spectrum of nutrients for optimal health.

b. Moderation and Mindful Eating

Understand the concept of mindful eating and how practicing moderation can foster a healthy relationship with food for the entire family.

CHAPTER 2

PLANNING FOR SUCCESS

Creating a healthy eating plan for your family involves thoughtful preparation and strategic planning. This chapter focuses on effective strategies to help you lay the groundwork for success in your journey toward healthier eating habits.

1. Setting Realistic Goals

a. Understanding Your Family's Needs and Preferences
Explore how to identify and consider the unique dietary needs and preferences of your family members when setting achievable health goals.
b. Establishing Realistic Milestones
Learn how to set incremental and achievable milestones to make progress toward long-term health goals without feeling overwhelmed.

2. Meal Planning Strategies

a. Benefits of Meal Planning

Understand the advantages of meal planning, including saving time, reducing food waste, and ensuring balanced nutrition for your family.

b. Creating a Meal Planning Routine

Discover practical tips and step-by-step guidance on how to create a meal-planning routine that suits your family's schedule and lifestyle.

3. Grocery Shopping Tips

a. Building a Healthy Shopping List

Learn how to compose a well-balanced shopping list that includes fresh produce, whole grains, lean proteins, and other essential items for nutritious meals.

b. Smart Shopping Habits

Explore strategies for navigating the grocery store, such as reading labels, selecting seasonal produce, and avoiding impulse purchases.

CHAPTER 3
BREAKFASTS FOR CHAMPIONS

Breakfast is the foundation of a healthy day and sets the tone for your family's energy and focus. In this chapter, we explore a variety of nutritious and delicious breakfast options that will fuel your family's mornings.

1. Energizing Breakfast Options

a. Power-Packed Protein Breakfasts
Discover protein-rich breakfast ideas that provide sustained energy and keep your family feeling full and satisfied throughout the morning.
b. Nutrient-Dense Breakfast Bowls and Smoothies
Explore creative and customizable breakfast bowl and smoothie recipes packed with essential vitamins and minerals.

2. Quick and Nutritious Morning Meals

a. On-the-Go Breakfasts

Find quick and easy breakfast solutions suitable for busy mornings, ensuring your family starts the day right, even when time is limited.

b. Make-Ahead Breakfasts for Convenience

Learn about make-ahead breakfast recipes that can be prepared in advance, simplifying your mornings without compromising on nutrition.

3. Grab-and-Go Breakfast Ideas

a. Portable Breakfast Snacks

Discover portable and nutritious breakfast snack ideas perfect for those mornings when your family needs a quick bite on the way out the door.

b. Breakfast Treats with a Healthy Twist

Explore healthier versions of classic breakfast treats, allowing your family to indulge without sacrificing nutritional value.

CHAPTER 4
LUNCHES ON THE GO

Lunchtime can be a challenging meal to plan, especially when you and your family are busy with work, school, or various activities. This chapter is dedicated to providing nutritious and convenient lunch options that can be enjoyed at home, school, or the workplace.

1. Packing Healthy Lunches for Work or School

a. Bento Box and Lunchbox Ideas

Explore creative and balanced lunchbox ideas suitable for both children and adults, ensuring a variety of nutrients in each meal.

b. Preparing Ahead for Packed Lunches

Learn about meal prep techniques and recipes that make packing nutritious lunches convenient and stress-free.

2. Balanced Lunchbox Ideas

: a. Sandwich and Wrap Varieties

Discover innovative and healthy sandwich and wrap recipes that go beyond the ordinary, incorporating a range of flavors and nutritious ingredients.

b. Salad Jars and Satisfying Salads

Explore the concept of salad jars and nutritious salad options that are both filling and flavorful, perfect for on-the-go lunches.

3. Simple Lunchtime Solutions

a. Soups, Stews, and One-Pot Meals

Find easy-to-make soups, stews, and one-pot meals that can be prepared in advance and reheated for a hassle-free lunch.

b. Leftovers Reinvented

Learn creative ways to repurpose leftovers from dinner into exciting and delicious lunch options for the next day.

CHAPTER 5

WHOLESOME DINNERS FOR THE FAMILY

Dinnertime offers an opportunity for families to come together and enjoy a nourishing meal. This chapter focuses on providing delicious and nutritious dinner options that are family-friendly, easy to prepare, and perfect for busy weeknights.

1. Easy Weeknight Dinner Recipes

a. Quick and Simple Dinners

Explore recipes that can be prepared in under 30 minutes, allowing you to serve a wholesome meal without spending excessive time in the kitchen.

b. Sheet Pan and One-Pot Meals

Discover the convenience of sheet pan and one-pot meals that minimize cleanup while maximizing flavor and nutrition.

2. One-Pot Meals for Busy Evenings

a. Casseroles and Oven-Baked Dishes

Explore hearty and comforting casseroles and oven-baked dishes that are perfect for feeding the whole family with minimal effort.

b. Slow Cooker and Instant Pot Creations

Learn about slow cooker and Instant Pot recipes that simplify dinner preparation, allowing flavors to meld while you attend to other tasks.

3. Family-Friendly Healthy Dinners

a. Kid-Friendly Meals

Find recipes tailored to appeal to children's tastes while still providing essential nutrients for their growth and development.

b. Balancing Taste and Nutrition

Discover strategies for incorporating healthy ingredients into family-favorite dishes without sacrificing flavor.

CHAPTER 6

SNACK ATTACKS MADE HEALTHY

Snacks play a significant role in maintaining energy levels and preventing overeating during meals. This chapter focuses on providing nutritious snack options that are satisfying, delicious, and suitable for all ages.

1. Nutritious Snack Choices for All Ages

a. Fruits, Vegetables, and Dips

Explore creative ways to incorporate fruits and vegetables into snacks, accompanied by delicious and healthy dip options.

b. Nut and Seed Snack Ideas

Discover nutritious and protein-packed snack ideas using various nuts, seeds, and their combinations.

2. Creating Snack Stations

a. Organizing Healthy Snack Stations

Learn how to set up snack stations in your home, encouraging healthier choices for both kids and adults.

b. DIY Snack Mixes and Trail Mixes

Explore customizable snack mix recipes that allow you to control ingredients and cater to your family's preferences.

3. Snack Prep and Portion Control

a. Batch Snack Preparation

Discover batch preparation techniques that make it easier to have healthy snacks readily available throughout the week.

b. Portion Control Strategies

Learn about portion control techniques and serving sizes to ensure balanced snacking without overindulging.

CHAPTER 7

DESSERTS WITH A HEALTHIER TWIST

Desserts can be delicious without compromising on nutrition. This chapter focuses on providing satisfying sweet treats that incorporate healthier ingredients, allowing your family to indulge guilt-free.

1. Guilt-Free Sweet Treats

a. Fruit-Based Desserts

Explore dessert recipes centered around fresh fruits, offering sweetness and natural goodness.

b. Yogurt and Frozen Treats

Discover recipes for frozen desserts and yogurt-based treats that provide a refreshing and healthier alternative to traditional sweets.

2. Dessert Hacks for Healthier Indulgences

a. Baking with Healthier Ingredients

Learn about substitutions and alternative ingredients to create healthier versions of classic baked desserts.

b. Reduced-Sugar Dessert Options

Explore recipes that use less refined sugars or natural sweeteners without compromising on taste.

3. Satisfying the Sweet Tooth

a. Portion-Controlled Desserts

Discover dessert options that come in individual portions, promoting moderation and mindful eating.

b. Desserts Rich in Nutrients

Explore recipes that incorporate nutritious ingredients such as nuts, seeds, and whole grains into sweet treats.

CHAPTER 8

SPECIAL OCCASIONS AND CELEBRATIONS

Maintaining a healthy eating plan doesn't mean sacrificing joyous moments. This chapter focuses on navigating special occasions, holidays, and celebrations while making mindful choices and balancing indulgence with nutritious options.

1. Healthy Party Planning

a. Planning Healthier Party Menus

Explore strategies for creating party menus that incorporate healthier options without compromising on taste and enjoyment.

b. Smart Substitutions and Recipe Makeovers

Learn about ingredient substitutions and recipe makeovers to transform traditional party favorites into healthier alternatives.

2. Holiday Eating Tips

a. Healthy Holiday Traditions

Discover ways to establish new, health-conscious traditions during holiday seasons and celebrations.

b. Mindful Eating During Festivities

Explore mindful eating practices to help your family make conscious choices while enjoying festive meals.

3. Balancing Treats and Healthy Choices

a. Moderation During Celebrations

Learn strategies for managing portion sizes and balancing indulgent treats with healthier meal choices during special occasions.

b. Encouraging Active Celebrations

Explore ways to incorporate physical activities or fun games into celebrations, promoting an active lifestyle alongside food enjoyment.

CHAPTER 9

STAYING ON TRACK

Consistency is key to maintaining a healthy eating plan. This chapter focuses on addressing challenges, maintaining Motivation, and celebrating progress to sustain a wholesome approach to family nutrition.

1. Overcoming Challenges in Eating Healthy

a. Addressing Common Obstacles

Explore strategies for overcoming common hurdles, such as time constraints, picky eaters, or conflicting schedules that may disrupt healthy eating habits.

b. Handling Cravings and Temptations

Learn techniques to manage cravings and navigate temptations without derailing your family's commitment to a nutritious eating plan.

2. Maintaining Motivation

a. Setting and Reviewing Goals

Explore the importance of setting achievable goals and periodically reviewing them to stay motivated on your family's health journey.

b. Encouraging Family Participation

Discover ways to involve family members in meal planning and preparation, fostering a sense of shared responsibility and Motivation.

3. Celebrating Progress and Success

a. Recognizing Milestones

Learn the significance of acknowledging and celebrating small achievements along the way to maintaining a positive mindset.

b. Reinforcing Healthy Habits

Explore methods to reinforce healthy eating habits within the family, creating a sustainable and lasting lifestyle change.

CONCLUSION

Congratulations on completing " Conquer Your Diet: The Healthy Cookbook for a Family Eating Plan"! This journey toward embracing nutritious eating habits for your family has been a valuable step toward fostering a healthier lifestyle.

1. Final Thoughts on Sustainable Healthy Eating

a. Embracing a Healthier Lifestyle

Reflect on the positive changes made throughout this book and how they've contributed to your family's overall well-being.

b. Building Sustainable Habits

Reinforce the importance of maintaining the healthy eating habits and routines established, emphasizing their long-term benefits.

2. Tips for Continuing the Journey

a. Consistency and Flexibility

Highlight the significance of consistency in healthy eating while allowing flexibility to accommodate life's changes and challenges.

b. Continuing Education and Exploration

Encourage ongoing exploration of new recipes, ingredients, and strategies to keep family meals exciting and diverse.

3. Thank You and Best Wishes

a. Acknowledging Family Efforts

Express gratitude for the commitment and effort your family has put into embracing a healthier eating plan.

b. Wishing for Continued Health and Wellness

Extend well wishes for continued success on your family's journey toward better health and vitality through mindful eating.

Closing Remarks

Conclusion: This book marks not just the end of a chapter but the beginning of a new, healthier lifestyle for your family. By prioritizing nutritious and delicious meals, you've laid the foundation for sustained health and happiness. Remember, every step taken toward healthier eating habits is a step toward a brighter, more energetic future for your loved ones.

Thank you for joining us on this journey to better health through mindful and nutritious eating!